GOOD VIBRATIONS
Clearing spaces and creating harmony

GOOD VIBRATIONS
Clearing spaces and creating harmony

By Maureen Williams
with Christine Day

ATHENA PRESS
LONDON

GOOD VIBRATIONS
Clearing spaces and creating harmony
Copyright © Maureen Williams 2006

All Rights Reserved

No part of this book may be reproduced in any form
by photocopying or by any electronic or mechanical means,
including information storage and retrieval systems,
without permission in writing from both the copyright
owner and the publisher of this book.

ISBN 1 84401 691 9

First Published 2006 by
ATHENA PRESS
Queen's House, 2 Holly Road
Twickenham TW1 4EG
United Kingdom

Printed for Athena Press

ABOUT THE AUTHORS

MAUREEN WILLIAMS, palmist, graphologist and counsellor, is well known for her readings and gifted teaching. In *Good Vibrations*, Maureen talks to the writer Christine Day about her groundbreaking healing work clearing negative energies with the pendulum, in which she now specialises.

CHRISTINE DAY, writer, artist and journalist, has written a number of books and her work has appeared in numerous magazines and newspapers. She agreed to collaborate on *Good Vibrations* after Maureen successfully cleared negative energies in her home.

INTRODUCTION

THIS BOOK describes my background in psychic work, and gradual move into the world of dowsing. From initially being interested in the whole area, I was eventually drawn to help people who seemed to have difficulties with themselves, their partners or homes, which could not be dealt with by traditional methods.

The negative influences from discarnate beings, as well as geopathic stress, is addressed through a combination of pendulum dowsing and an ability to intuitively understand in some detail what is going on in a person's life. Therefore, once the problem is cleared through transference of energy to the client, that person can take control of their life again and make whatever changes are necessary.

Several examples of various 'clearings' I have carried out are documented and can be authenticated.

Please visit my website at www.goodvibrations.eu.com.

Maureen Williams

CONTENTS

Beginnings	12
Poltergeists	16
My Move to Brighton	18
My Homespun Philosophy	21
Some of my Experiences	26
Some Thoughts on Exorcism	32
Asking For and Receiving Help	38
Mysterious Happenings	41
Procedures	44
Rescuing the Living	50
Hauntings	56
A Curse	65
The Dominatrix	69
Automatic Writing	72
Sisters	74
A Musician	75
Guilty Hormones	78
Electrical Rays	79
A Widow	80
Black Energy	82
Imprints	84
A Fine Line	88

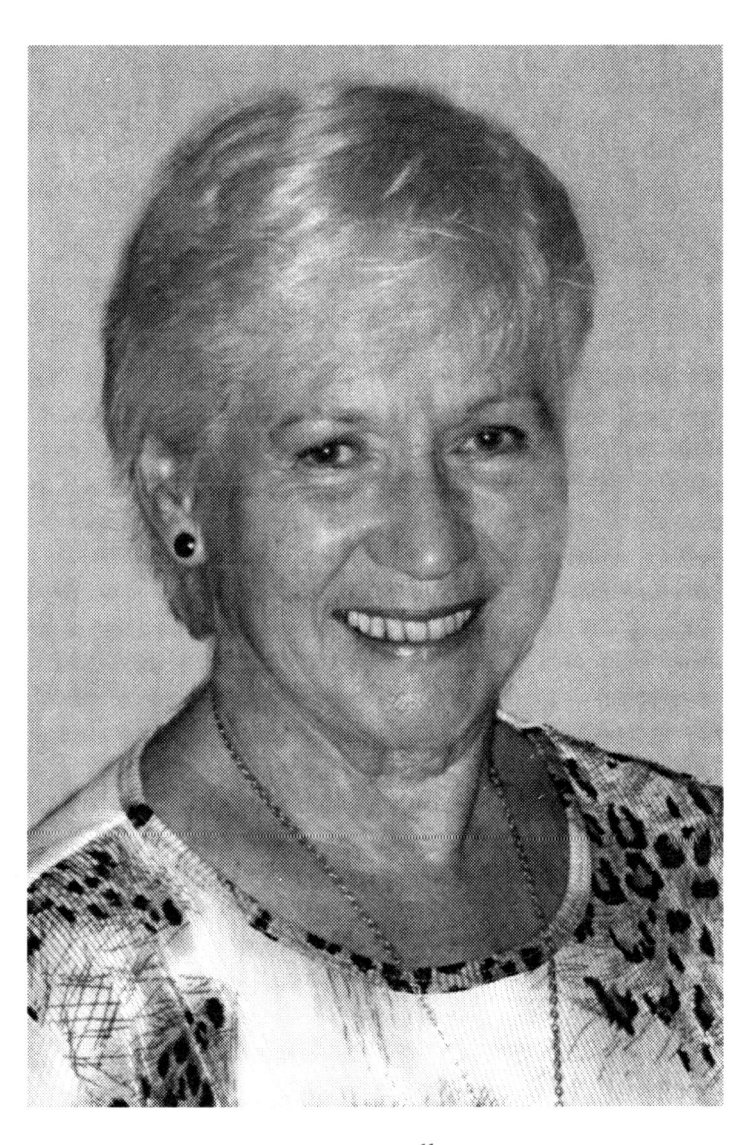

Maureen Williams

BEGINNINGS

MY MOTHER had a severe nervous breakdown when I was twelve, and although I had no knowledge or understanding of this condition, the experience was an initiation into adult emotional problems. Her personality changed, and to me, as a child, her behaviour was unrecognisable – but nobody seemed to know the real reason why, and that unanswered question occupied most of my waking (and sometimes sleeping) hours for the next two years, until she recovered. In those days, the Forties, prescription drugs for severe depression were not generally used, and after two years of misery for my mother and indeed the whole family, she had electrical treatment.

But it was the first of many breakdowns. I think I looked into these things more deeply than the average child of my age and was very sensitive to everyone's reactions. It seemed clear to me that her breakdown was mainly connected with her family background. She was the youngest in a large, close-knit Irish family, and was much loved and protected, and very innocent. She had very little defence against the world, and when issues came up in her life that required emotional strength, she couldn't cope.

As a young child, I was clairvoyant in the sense of being able to see many figures around me who seemed to inhabit my bedroom. I had a huge Egyptian standing by the door. I can see him now, standing there with his spear. There was also an Indian and a Chinaman. They were comforting. We didn't communicate, they were just there. Sometimes I used to shut my eyes, but they were there even with my eyes shut. They were probably there to watch over me. I felt protected, but never felt the need to tell anyone about them. It was wartime. There were difficulties, stresses and strains in the family, and that's probably why these Spirits appeared. I was anxious because my mother wasn't well, and perplexed because there was nothing that could be done to alter the situation. Her hair fell out and she used to walk around singing and muttering, seemingly living in another world.

This went on for nearly two years. My mother was in her mid-thirties, and so, since she was in a happy marriage with two much-loved children, one had to go back over the years for the trigger, which was not really obvious. Her breakdown seemed to have been precipitated by the sudden death of my grandmother, who was living with us at the time. I don't think anyone realised how important her mother was to her. In a very big family, my grandmother was very much the matriarch. As soon as my mother married, she put the pressure on my grandmother to come and live with her, along with one of her sisters. Mother was very happy with my father but was obviously used to having her family around. This was during World War II, and tragically my grandmother died of a heart attack in the Shelter in the middle of an air raid. This was very traumatic for the family, and particularly we children, as we were all in the Shelter at the time. Subsequently, my mother's sister, who was also living with us, moved away because we children were getting older and needed our own rooms. At this point, my poor mother went into a really bad breakdown, recounted above, and this tendency stayed with her for the rest of her life. She had several more serious breakdowns; eventually she was permanently on a cocktail of drugs for twenty years. She had been very dependent on her mother's strength and protection – a lesson I learnt at that early age, which has helped me to be comfortably independent for many years now.

I learnt a great deal from this experience, and my work has subsequently involved helping people with problems that I have experienced myself. The spiritual element was always around me, but stayed 'on hold' for a long time. I was drawn to supernatural occurrences, and terribly keen to read and find out about them. I was particularly interested in palm reading, and also places that were haunted. Although I never knowingly experienced any *bad* energy during my early childhood, I expect there was a lot around, and I was fascinated by Spirits.

During the late Sixties and early Seventies I worked for the owner of Buxted Park Health Hydro, a Mrs Heather Shipman. She was very interested in spiritualism and entertained mediums there. At the time, she was promoting and sponsoring an amateur pianist who played music channelled from famous composers such as Beethoven, Chopin and Liszt, and who subsequently performed at the Royal Albert Hall.

The pianist, Rosemary Brown, was a member of the Spiritualist Church and played the piano as a hobby. One day, quite unexpectedly, a figure appeared beside her, dressed in old-fashioned clothes, and announced himself as the composer Liszt. He asked her to write down some musical notes. She wrote them down and played them back. When they discovered she was a good 'channel', other famous, long-dead composers started coming through, and she was eventually inundated with new compositions by these old masters. Despite obvious scepticism, the musical compositions were never disproved, to my knowledge, and this was a great eye-opener to me. The concert was a great success.

I was working with this element for the first time, and the whole time spent with Mrs Shipman was a kind of entrée into the world of mediumship.

Later, in the late Seventies, I fully developed my palm

reading and also taught myself graphology. These skills don't appear, on the surface, to be very spiritual, but they were my way of tuning into people's lives. Eventually I gave up all aspects of office life and trained as a counsellor. I also studied tarot and joined a circuit of psychic readers going round London working at Psychic Fairs. Although I never publicise myself as a tarot reader, I find the cards very helpful to use after a palm reading when I am 'tuned in'. It enables me to see what is going on in a person's life, then and there.

I had always realised that Spirits were just disembodied people, and that's why I wasn't afraid. I think they made themselves known to me when I was small because of the difficult situation at home. Of course, I'm no longer in that state of mind; there's nobody around me causing a troubled atmosphere. But often at night, in the darkness of my bedroom, I see shadows and sense, rather than see, the Egyptian with his spear! In the darkness, I sometimes see faces moving in a strange sort of way, floating in space. One will come forward and I'll be able to see it very clearly. When I was a child I didn't know how to deal with this. I used to say: 'Go away, I want to go to sleep.' Then I realised I had to be very firm and tell them categorically to go and not come back. I might or might not have spoken out loud. I certainly learnt to use these positive thoughts. I wasn't saying 'Please', I was actually telling Spirits who were intrusive to go. It seems to me now that I was preparing to do the work of clearing Spirits.

POLTERGEISTS

In 1991 I visited the United States, and when I returned to my flat in London's Docklands, which had been occupied by tenants for over two years, I had a very disturbing experience. My tenants had left the place in a mess and my heart sank when I moved back in. They handed over the keys at midday and then went off. In the evening, I heard this terrific crash and discovered that a large wall mirror had come off its hook and smashed on the floor. Then, the following day, a very big picture came crashing down and hit a table, breaking the frame and glass. Then a smaller picture fell from the wall. This was happening in different areas of the flat, and went on for several days. Quickly realising that something abnormal was happening, I became really scared.

I was in a bit of a state because the tenants had left me with various items of maintenance to repair. The problem continued, and I began to think I had a poltergeist in the flat. I couldn't think of anything else it could be. I didn't know who to turn to. Whatever it was induced a great deal of fear in me because it was violent. Then a friend came to stay with me for a couple of days, and on her departure I drove her back to London Bridge station. When I came back to the flat, a very heavy storage heater had become unhinged and was hanging off the wall! At this point, I really had the jitters. I said my prayers and begged it to stop. I contacted a woman who dealt with manifestations of this kind and left a message on her answering machine, but she didn't phone back. This increased my desperation. I was so keyed up that I knelt down in the middle of my living room and said: *'Go away, in the name of God. You're not wanted here. I never want this to happen again!'*

I was very positive and I cleared it with this performance. But it gave me first-hand knowledge of this kind of experience, which has proved invaluable. Not long after this strange experience I began learning, through channelling energy, to help people with similar problems. And the pendulum became my tool – and my new friend.

MY MOVE TO BRIGHTON

I MOVED to Brighton, in East Sussex, in 1994 and met Jim Ives, a healer who was interested in dowsing. He was using his pendulum over special symbols to effect a clearing of negative forces, and as I was going through a prolonged period of extreme tiredness, he offered to visit me, using the pendulum to gauge the geopathic stress in my flat. He found an excess of electrical rays there, which my body had absorbed, and advised me to put a special symbol over the electricity meter. Afterwards, I felt much better and was most impressed.

We became very good friends. I knew how to dowse, but these symbols opened up the healing and clearing aspect of this technique. We both work with vibrations to discover what is causing problems. This can be Spirits, underground water, radar rays, electric rays or illness, to name a few causes. Each has a different vibration. Our bodies also have a vibration. If we are attacked by something which has a different vibration from our own, we react and it unsettles us.

Although most people are familiar with the dowsing rods used for finding water (and all manner of other geological matter besides), most will not realise that an experienced dowser holding a pendulum can obtain the same answers, and more, than with a rod. The pendulum is a finding tool, and it can be anything from a ring on a string to an expensive crystal on a silver chain. And it appears to give you the answer whatever you ask, providing the answer can be provided by swinging in a clockwise or anticlockwise direction – *yes* or *no* to your question. Your mind must be clear, your questions well-intentioned, with no personal gain – and behold, once the pendulum has gained your trust, it is truly reliable. The brain seems to house knowledge which its owner doesn't know exists, and the pendulum's swing – quite independent of its owner – obliges with the answer to most of the questions put to it. Some people have a greater affinity with the pendulum than others, and intuition and practise play a large part. But pendulum dowsing has never been scientifically explained. All we dowsers can say is – it works!

I use a mixture of symbols and charts channelled by other healers and have developed my own system, which is very simplified, to clear unwanted energy from people and their personal spaces – even animals. I swing the pendulum over the symbol I have selected and ask my Higher Self to clear the energy, or to take a Spirit to the Light. I always prepare myself beforehand with a prayer, and never work on any subject I am not certain about. The pendulum provides me with most of my answers and information that I can pass on to my client. The effect is usually immediate.

Jim was doing a lot of research into various symbols, and passed on his knowledge to me. I loved these symbols, and started using the pendulum over them to create a healing energy which I myself could use. Because of my interest in these matters, people started telling me that there was something wrong with their house, or a particular room, and I began dowsing to determine which symbols I needed to use to resolve the problem. This was the start of the healing work I am doing today.

I now specialise in clearing negative energies. These can come from the earth, sky, bricks and mortar, or an entity of some description, a discarnate. Negativity can have a detrimental long-term influence on a person's health and their state of mind.

I'm very practical in the way I approach people, yet I work very intuitively. I tend to use two symbols, and find out from dowsing, using a question and answer technique, exactly what is wrong with a client and why they are being troubled. If the latent problem lies with geopathic or electrical rays, they may have to change certain things in the home. Sometimes this is impossible and the only thing a person can do is move.

I firmly believe that our Spirit moves on to other planes of existence when we die. Many people who have died in tragic circumstances or have not led very good lives leave their Spirit in what we call limbo or purgatory. These discarnates don't belong on this earth plane, but haven't found their next destination. They tend to hone in on atmospheres with which they were familiar when in human form. For example, very often somebody who drinks heavily or who takes drugs has discarnates around him who also had these addictions.

MY HOMESPUN PHILOSOPHY

I FEEL very strongly driven to do this work. For most of my life, I have had problems with electrical equipment malfunctioning around me, and I have been advised in the past by various psychics that I should be 'channelling' (or using) this very strong magnetic energy. I didn't really understand what they meant, but now I realise that with my current work I am channelling it in a constructive and beneficial way.

The people who have psychic problems tend to be those who are very sensitive. Of course, more and more people are realising that you can be influenced by your environment because of the interest in Feng Shui, where you rearrange the furniture and put plants (for example) in certain parts of the home to transform the energy. With my work I don't actually change the energy. I eliminate certain energies and allow the positive to take over again.

I sometimes advise people to sleep in different rooms. They are quite happy moving things around in their living room, but it's amazing how reticent they can be about moving their bedroom. Often there can be something very disturbing going on in a bedroom, especially at night. A typical experience can be that of feeling somebody lying down beside you on the bed. I've experienced that myself, several times, but I didn't know how to deal with it in those days. Sometimes, even if you clear the room of Spirits, a person is on overload and it is advisable for them to sleep in another room for a few days, even weeks, before going back to sleep again in their own room.

If people are sensitive, they are generally open to experiencing problems of this kind, but also open to being helped. When clients relate their peculiar experiences, they want to know why they are going through these things, and listen to my explanations even if, initially, they don't believe in them wholeheartedly. It is all a question of understanding that we are not without influences beyond the human realm – not an easy explanation to accept.

My clients are very often people to whom I've given readings, or friends. I run groups and workshops and often explain my 'clearing technique'. It registers in the minds of my clients and students, and so people are recommended to me. It's amazing how it gets about! A friend, or client, might just happen to voice that they feel they've got something really negative dragging them down all the time. They don't know what it is, but very often it is this burden of negative spiritual energy, or a disembodied Spirit, that is having a most negative effect on that person. When you rid them of it they feel amazingly better. It's like the sun coming out from behind the clouds.

It seems to be acknowledged by many people that it is a natural progression for our Spirits to go on somewhere after death. So many who come back from a near-death experience report that they seemed to be going down a tunnel with white light at the end. I feel that the body is just a temporary house for the soul. If someone dies in an accident or in sudden circumstances, they haven't made preparations for their death. Often the body dies but the Spirit stays. The Spirit often wants to be where it used to be, but the earth plane is no longer the right place for the Spirit to be. What I always ask is that the Spirit goes to its right and proper place. I don't judge whether it's been a good person in the human form, because that's not in my domain. But you let it know that you can release it and ask if it would like to be released. The Spirit will nearly always say '*Yes*' and go.

There are thousands and thousands of Spirits in this lost state. Certainly, lack of preparation seems to be part of the problem. As a Catholic, I remember that there is a special prayer for a peaceful death. To make the transit from death to the afterlife, it is important to feel secure in the belief that, although you don't know what is going to happen to you when you die, you are spiritually prepared. When you don't have this opportunity, there are often repercussions.

Spirits take energy from the people they are close to and from surroundings. If they are attached to a person, or around a person, it creates a dark cloud. If it's an actual attachment, which means the person is almost possessed, a lot of the person's own natural personality is being taken away. This doesn't happen that often, but when it does, it is serious.

I think that many of the people who are in mental hospitals are in some form of possession by discarnates with a very negative energy around them. They are diagnosed as schizophrenics because they are acting completely out of context with their own personality. I have successfully healed people with discarnates around them, who have been considered schizophrenic because their whole personality has been suppressed. The daughter of one particular client couldn't communicate with her family at all. She was completely dislocated from life and was in a mental institution. She was diagnosed as schizophrenic and was hearing voices. Once I had cleared the bad energy, she was allowed home by the consultant within a few days. Her mother, who had asked me to help, said she at last had her daughter back, and was so happy. The girl's problem resulted from a car accident which had led to deep depression – then voices.

People do often attract Spirits when they are at a low ebb.

If you are gaily and optimistically going about your life, you shouldn't have these problems. But if there is something not right and there is some negativity around you or within you, perhaps even in parents, partners or children, then this attracts the wrong energies to you, which can on occasion wreak havoc.

It is possible to see a Programme in someone's life, just as you have a program in a computer. These Programmes are inbuilt characteristics, which are hard to break. The Programmes I dowse for include Greed, Envy, Cowardice, Failure, Escapism – and many more. If people do have a particular Programme which they have not worked at removing, then it is likely that whatever Spirit is around them will have had those particular traits. You'll find that if someone you know is a drinker, for example, then most of their friends are drinkers too. They don't want to be with someone who is teetotal because that makes them feel uncomfortable. I feel that, likewise, earthbound Spirits actually gravitate to what they are used to, and if you get rid of the Spirit you can very often lift the person out of that Programme. Otherwise, they become embedded in it.

Some people are aware that they have an entity with them – but others are not. It very much depends on the person. I think it is quite a scary fact that when I'm giving help to people I have to judge for myself whether I'm going to divulge whether it's a Spirit or not. I'm more inclined to say it is negative energy. If they really want to delve into it I will say that possibly it's a discarnate and I'll begin to explain my philosophy. But if they don't want to go deeply into it, I won't. Discarnates often have a negative energy, but the term 'negative energy' can apply to other things in the home as well, including geopathic stress.

The presence of discarnates can go far back into the past and they may have not necessarily been around just one person. A Spirit doesn't have to have had any relationship with the person it attaches to. It could even be a soldier from World War I who was killed in action, for example, with absolutely no connection with the person concerned. There's no such thing as time in the world of Spirit – or so I believe.

SOME OF MY EXPERIENCES

IF IT'S A property with a problem, I might not have to investigate the circumstances that surround it. But if it affects a person, I tend to be more interested in the reasons why, and delve. Some people do have horrible experiences, particularly that of being held down in bed at night. I remember experiencing that a lot as a child – feeling this weight and not being able to move. There is also the experience of having something lying beside you.

I'm helping a woman at the moment who has 'visitations'. I'm inclined to believe that these experiences are not just down to her imagination, because I've had similar experiences myself. Way back, I went away for a romantic weekend with my husband and we stayed at a very old inn called Who'd Have Thought It? in Devon. The room had sloping floorboards and a huge four-poster bed. When we went to bed, I could feel something depressing the mattress on *my* side. I turned over, but knew it was still there. I stayed like that for a long time, not terrified exactly, but very uncomfortable with the situation. I felt in a frozen state. I wanted to go to the bathroom but couldn't move. Eventually, I plucked up the courage and stepped over John, not wanting to go the other side where this 'thing' was lying. When I came back, the presence had gone!

In the morning there was a little book on the breakfast

table explaining the history of the place. The room was haunted by a knight who, in the olden days, had come back to seek his lady love. If I had not known this, I might have tended to go along with the psychiatrists and think it was only my imagination. But, historically, so many people had had the same experience in that room, and I'd experienced it without knowing the history. I told John. He was totally noncommittal, as usual, although he didn't tell me not to talk rubbish!

Once, I was staying with a friend whose house was part of an old monastery near Rye. I was looking after the dogs whilst she was away and was given a very old room with heavy beams. As I fell into sleep, I felt this incredibly heavy weight on me, pushing me, pinning me down. It seemed to be over my face as well. After feeling this sensation for some time, and feeling quite panicky, I adamantly told whatever it was to '*Go in the name of God.*' I was released – perhaps from the spiritual presence of an unhappy monk! I got up and turned on a wall light and left it on. I stayed there for another two weeks, but there were no more problems.

Our senses vary a great deal, and that's why, if there is something around, one person can gauge its presence – it may be on their wavelength – and another can't. Some people can smell perfume or cigar smoke; others don't notice it.

I was never comfortable in the house we lived in at Bromley. We moved there when I was fifteen. It was much larger than the previous house, and everyone else loved it. But there was one room I couldn't bear to go into – an extra room built above the garage. When I married, at twenty-one years of age, I moved up to Scotland to start a new life, and after about five years we moved back temporarily to the Bromley house with two children and a dog. We were staying, in fact, with my parents while we were house-hunting, my husband having been relocated to London. I ended up sleeping in the room I had always hated passing on my way downstairs during the night! It still felt creepy. But nobody else was bothered and I had to grin and bear the discomfort that sleeping in that room caused me. I wish I knew then what I know now! I think something very sad had happened in that room and left a residue of unhappiness.

One of the things that can really leave a residue in a place is a Ouija board. You can have a really nice group of people who decide to use a Ouija board and they might only use it once, but certain Spirits can be drawn in that linger and taint the atmosphere. Someone who is really sensitive can pick up that something is still there. I'm truly anti Ouija boards. Friends of mine still use them when they want an answer to a problem. I think it's the wrong way to try to get answers, and certainly Spirits should not be used for 'a bit of fun'! I don't think this 'pastime' attracts good Spirits. They might say they are your mother, or your old uncle, but there is no proof. And what discarnate of any calibre would resort to giving answers to people looking for a cheap thrill? I really don't believe that you can completely rely on Spirits to give you information in this way. I prefer to stick to my intuition and what seems to be a direct line to my Higher Self.

Sometimes when giving readings, or dowsing, I see pictures. I don't often hear voices. I tend to have a vision, or feel a sensation. I certainly don't start dowsing and expect to see a picture. My method is to ask questions and answers over a wide range of things, through the pendulum. I've got charts which I use to gauge, measure and if possible define the problem given to me by a client, and if there is a Spirit present, I ask what kind it is. You can gauge anything – from the really transient sort (which is completely harmless), to the Spirits that make me quite uncomfortable to have around. And there are those in between. I find out what intensity they are (how strong their presence, or influence, is) by grading from one to ten. If I discover a Spirit's intensity is

SOME OF MY EXPERIENCES

three or under, then it is on the light side and much easier to clear. This kind of Spirit is just a lost soul – in the wrong space – just waiting for some help to go to its rightful place. This work is so necessary, as it seems that so many souls do not pass over easily, and need prayers and other forms of help to move them on.

Anything that I want to know – providing it is a yes or no answer – the pendulum will tell me. I have no idea how this kind of dowsing actually works, but to be a good dowser you have to have a totally clear mind. If you've got a personal problem yourself at that time, or are lacking concentration, or, even more important, have an emotional link with your client, you're not going to get the true picture. This is why I like doing this work anonymously. I use the same technique as in my graphology work where I analyse people's handwriting. The less you know about a person to start with, the more you are able to find out for yourself in a completely impartial way. When my head is totally clear and I have no prior knowledge, I'm going to get a completely objective result. My method gives me figures and information about how weak or how strong an energy is and how many years it has been around. I'm tuning in and building up a picture. I don't rely completely on psychic ability such as clairvoyance or mediumship; my method is more of an investigation, testing the energy and moving it on.

I don't talk to the Spirits, except to ask them – through my Higher Self – if they are willing to go. (This way, I am protected from dealing with discarnates at first hand.) Everything else I can find out from the pendulum. People are very fascinated when they get the results of my findings (which I always record and file) and they can often relate their difficulties to an explanation I give them about the existence of 'Programmes'. These Programmes are blocks, or personality problems – Abuse or Jealousy, for instance – and can be something they have experienced in their lives or

SOME OF MY EXPERIENCES

from people around them. They understand that their own personal problems are often encouraging that Spirit to hang around. (Of course, there are those other Spirits which are harmless and readily go. They don't play havoc with people's lives.)

The more outrageous or the more unusual a 'happening' is, its very occurrence helps people to accept that my investigations might hold the explanation. If someone has a serious problem in their home and/or their personal life, which eases off when I have done my work, these clients are converted in all cases. But I tend not to give too many explanations of how I work because for the uninitiated (spiritually) it is not easy to understand these things.

In the early days, I didn't expect anyone who had asked for help to confirm that everything was clear – sometimes I even phoned them up afterwards to ask if it was all right because I needed to know. Now, part of the deal is that they do need to let me know, every step of the way: if an energy has only partly gone or if it gets worse – things often have to get worse before they get better! – I might have cleared one thing and left an opening for something else. On a few occasions when I'm clearing, a person is so open that they are very vulnerable still and something else will crop up. That is not a reflection on my work because I am doing whatever is needed at the time. I endeavour to 'close people down', by spiritual healing and protection, but it's really something they have to be prepared to do themselves. Some people walk around all the time totally open to 'otherworldliness'. The sort of person whose mother is always upsetting them, or the father, or the children, also tend to take on board whatever negative energy is around them and never close down. These people often get interference from Spirits. You clear them spiritually and, three months later, they need clearing again! I can balance the chakras (the chakras are a kind of spiritual energy system which, in a healthy person, are in balance) but they will open again because of a person's genetic disposition. You can help someone but you can't change them. For example, if somebody has very dry hair that is unmanageable, you can put conditioner on and it looks absolutely beautiful. But directly their hair is washed, it's the same as before! This applies to healing. In general, I think healing has been misunderstood; people believe that by having healing everything's going to improve. Well, it helps at that particular point, but there are so many ingredients in a person's life that just receiving healing doesn't last unless the person changes. *How you live your life is so important in all this.*

And also, the state of mind in which you die! It is not desirable to die with spiritual negativity still around you or within you. Regression is considered by some to be quite dangerous because of what you might be bringing into the present. If you are regressed by a medium who doesn't understand the forces he or she is dealing with, this could be bringing up a lot of negative influence into the client's current existence.

I look to see what is bothering a person. If it's more than one discarnate, then how many – one, two, three, four, five, six? As I've mentioned, there are different grades of intensity – one to ten. With dowsing you can discover the intensity and also how long this energy has been there. The thing to do is to make the healing and clearing as simple as possible, and my way of working does not make things seem complicated. I'm really pleased if my healing has worked for a person, rather like a doctor finding the right remedy. I see myself in that category – I don't claim to have amazing gifts, and can teach anyone how to do this work if they have a genuine desire to help distressed people.

SOME THOUGHTS ON EXORCISM

EXORCISM TENDS to conjure up the scenario of having something terribly evil inside which is going to manifest in some way as it leaves the body. That's the impression we receive from horror films, and certainly it happens in real life too – but, fortunately, not too often!

I honestly have never had any experience like that, but I know there have been some clients who definitely had some kind of evil within them. Although it hasn't completely taken them over so that it needs total exorcism, it has had to be removed for them to live a normal life again. This seems to come out in people who are very weak or open, or those with deep depression or mental illness. There are people who probably have not even realised that they've been in an evil environment or been exposed to something very evil that has taken them over.

That might be as simple as being in bad company. If you are with people who are using or dealing drugs, there's a lot of bad energy which goes with the territory. If you are vulnerable at the time, this is when it is possible for a discarnate energy to take over. So major excesses such as drugs and drink – which can be mind-altering and cause someone to lose the sense of their own identity – can be real problems.

I'm sure it is possible for some people to have real personality changes in these circumstances, and may believe their

SOME THOUGHTS ON EXORCISM

own bad habits are responsible. But with those bad habits very often comes the spiritually negative side where discarnates are playing a part. Sometimes, for people in this state to be completely healed, they obviously need to dry out, kick the addiction and bad company, and if they can also get help of the type I give, it could assist their recovery.

If you suspect there is something really evil inside someone, you have to ask how it got there. It doesn't just happen. You have to investigate to see why this evil has manifested, and persists. This is a very important — but more unusual — side of my work.

I became sure when I had the poltergeist at my flat that something unpleasant had gone on there and left a negative spiritual residue. If we talk about 'Spirits', we conjure up a shape floating about and knocking the pictures down because we can't really comprehend the other world. It is easier to think of energy: if there is a very loud bang from a major explosion a mile away, our house might remain intact, but a picture might come off the wall. The sound produces an energy, a vibration, that could do that. That is how I think of energy. It's also what we create ourselves when we dash about. Of course, everything produces energy of some sort.

Most people have personality traits, often inherited. If you've got a balanced personality, you have an advantage. If you have a tendency towards Anger, for example, and it's balanced with a very positive trait like Kindness, then that's not so bad. But if something happens to make your Anger a very strong constituent of everyday life, and if something goes wrong at work or in the home and you're always angry, the positive traits seem to disappear. Then it's all about Anger, creating an extreme, and, energy-wise, you're definitely inviting a discarnate to join you in this negative state!

I sometimes wonder about people whose anger becomes violent — are they really becoming violent of their own volition or are they being encouraged by some negative

SOME THOUGHTS ON EXORCISM

force? It can't be proved either way, but if a person is genuinely trying to reform, they often seem to get spiritual help. If, however, you have something that is really rather negative in your personality, the trait can get worse if you don't seek that help.

It's really about boundaries and how far you go. Often we blame the Internet or television for carrying pornography and violence and believe this encourages people to carry out evil acts because they've been influenced by the media, etc. Experts are saying people could be totally addicted to *viewing* such things, but never *act* on it. So what actually makes someone take that big leap between *watching* and *acting out* evil deeds? We might feel that something does take them over, something very negative spiritually, without a doubt. These Spirits have lost their human boundaries, beyond which we average people don't normally go. So what force is driving us beyond the boundaries of acceptable behaviour to what people call evil? People 'dabble' sometimes in things they don't understand and get taken over by harmful energies. They can, for example, dabble in black magic or Voodoo and get out of their depth. It is quite possible that something evil may have taken over at that point to promote acts that appeal to our more bestial nature. I believe a satanic force takes over. Most people, even if they don't believe in Satan, know what that word infers. This is a very dark force behind an entity, which is urging on people who have lost their boundaries.

Don't forget, too, that Spirits can be harmless. That's why I have to investigate to see what category it falls into – to see if it's really going to cause havoc! It could be a Spirit just begging for help, release.

In the past, some mediums have told me I've still got the Spirit of my father around me, although in fact he's been dead for forty years. Some people, myself included, admit to feeling quite comfortable talking to their dead father, and

SOME THOUGHTS ON EXORCISM

feel he's really there. Well, if he really is there, and that's what is happening, then the whole scenario of life after death is opening up before our eyes – or, should I say, our senses! For example, if you leave the front door open, uninvited people can come in. So spiritually, if you leave the door open you never know who or what you're going to attract. Some clients complain about weird goings-on in their lives – something not very nice happening during the night, for instance, maybe something frightening – and then, during the daylight hours these people are often seeking communication with (perhaps through a medium) their father or mother (for example) who died many years ago. The cause of the problem is that these people are not *controlling* the situation, the door is ajar, and therefore at night time can attract the Spirits they *don't* want around them.

We *can* control the situation with Spirits. We have the power to allow them in or not. People feel powerless, but this is simply their perception – if you want to try to have some communication with the dead, go to a reputable medium. Otherwise, keep that spiritual door well and truly closed, just as you would lock your door at night. And be resolute about it.

I'm not really in favour of trying to communicate with Spirits who should really be helped to go to the Light. If the human form dies and its Spirit has gone to the right and proper place, one wonders if they should rest in peace and not be contacted to deliver sometimes very trivial messages. I personally don't think it's appropriate. When people first die I think they go into a limbo-like sphere. It is said that it takes a certain length of time for the Spirit to leave the earthly plane, and I think, during that period, if a medium wants to give comfort to somebody, that's fine. I would like to see it all left alone really. I've received messages from loved ones, usually through a medium, as many people have, but, philosophically, I think our own life is what we make it. If we really want spiritual help we turn to higher realms. If we

SOME THOUGHTS ON EXORCISM

call on the angels for help, that satisfies a spiritual need. When loved ones die and leave us without their love and care, the situation reminds me of a mother who goes out to work: she does her best to provide for her family's needs and then leaves the house. She doesn't keep running back!

When people die their Spirits are not really there to give in-depth advice. It is their 'essence' which has left the body behind and is on its natural journey onwards. Regarding mediumship, I think that certain Spirits communicate through a willing channel, but for some people these communications can go on for years and a certain dependency can form. Isn't it better just to let go? For a certain length of time when loved ones die you can glean a lot of comfort from receiving messages from them, or to just know they are still in contact. The natural process of bereavement is learning to let go. With the grieving, if you still feel they're around, you can still communicate with them in your head. That's fine. But beyond a reasonable time, consulting mediums to give you messages is not allowing that Spirit to move on.

The more mature and evolved you are, the more you are able to accept the period which is given to you for grieving, to have some kind of relationship with the departed in the process of grieving, and then, when it feels comfortable, let go. This is part of the natural grieving process. I personally have got to the point where my deceased loved ones are long gone and I'm very happy for them to be at peace where they are.

With my husband there was quite a tie after he died, even though our marriage had ended ten years previously. There were many messages from him, and in the end I really didn't want any more. If there has been a dependency on a person in life there can be a greater dependency on them when they are dead. We long for help and advice and to feel we are still loved. The way a person has felt for us never ever dies. That's a wonderful thing to know and experience, and death can make no difference to this knowledge. If you have a co-dependency, it's not going to break in death. It's a two-way need. My grandmother died when she was nearly eighty, and as I have outlined, it was almost impossible for some of the family to come to terms with her death. My mother (and my aunt to a lesser degree) had a breakdown. There was an unbreakable, and rather frightening, dependency on my grandmother being there. I've learnt a lot from seeing at first hand how devastating it is to lose someone as revered as that. I also do think, psychologically, the experience of death transforms us into the stuff we are made of. Some are more generously endowed with strength of character than others, and surviving bereavement is a proof of what we can do on our own. When all the chips are down, you are on your own! The one thing you don't want is anything around you that is going to impede your progress in life. One of the things I do feel very strongly is that hanging on to the past definitely impedes progress.

It's easier, freer, less restricting, not to be carrying the past. Some people are very private and one may mistakenly assume that their lives are running smoothly. But nobody knows, not even in the closest relationship, what's really going on in someone's thoughts. Out of really difficult personal events can emerge an opportunity to turn one's attention to a hitherto unnoticed milestone. Some of the best counsellors I know have had frantic lives themselves, but turned it around to benefit their work. Some people learn about Bereavement Counselling, start helping others in order to find a new raison d'etre in their lives, are even motivated to start charities which can benefit others, when their loved ones die tragically. This channels the energy and helps them move on in a positive way. But the path must always be stretching out before you, not turning back.

ASKING FOR AND RECEIVING HELP

I GET asked to help with all sorts of problems. For example, someone might phone me because something strange is going on at their office. Every time they go there they feel awful. Initially, I dowse to see if there is a problem where I can help. On two occasions the answer was *no* and I left it alone. I don't know the reason for this – it might have been to protect me. Mostly it is *yes*. Having written on a piece of paper the name and address of the client, I immediately check for geopathic stress. If there is a problem in this area I have to find out what is the root cause. This is by means of a *yes* or *no* swing of the pendulum. Then I'll ask if there's anything on a spiritual level affecting this person. It's like an investigation, carried out in a very personal and confidential way. I'm never cold or abstract. I want to know how to help the person; I always empathise, as only by understanding from my heart can I heal.

My will to make a bad situation better surges from my solar plexus and right through my body when I'm carrying out a clearing. The bigger the healing, the more important it is, the greater that feeling. It's not just the use of the pendulum, I feel a terrific desire and love for that person.

I do believe in the Higher Self – it seems to be another dimension of our spiritual self. It can be God. You have to go with what you believe. It does mean that if you ask for help

ASKING FOR AND RECEIVING HELP

you are not just doing it on your own. Because I have had a religious upbringing, I have always believed in different saints who can help us in different areas of our lives.

One particular saint who has recently been beatified is Padre Pio, and I've always really loved him. He went through crisis after crisis during his life. He was a modern priest who died in 1968 and became known for his healing powers. He had the stigmata (bleeding wounds on his hands and feet, replicating the wounds of Jesus on the cross) and scourge marks on his back. They appeared overnight when he was a young man, stayed with him until his death, and never stopped bleeding. When he was alive he was bi-locational. He might be saying Mass in Italy and appearing to a troubled person in America at the same time. This is something the Church tried not to comment on until his great healing powers got so much publicity that it had to be recognised. He has many devotees, including myself. He healed people wherever he went, and was greatly loved. Since his death, he has continued to appear to people in need. He is very accessible, even in death, and if you particularly want some help or guidance you can ask him to intercede for you and he does. They say if he is around you, you can smell the scent of roses. I've experienced this several times. For myself, I am no longer a practising Catholic, but I still have the 'faith'. I certainly believe in the life, death and resurrection of Jesus, but I simply cannot approve of the authoritarian and unbending nature of the Catholic Church. I practise on my own terms, and don't feel under any obligation to 'toe the line' as a Catholic. However, much of the doctrine is incredibly spiritual and has played a major part in my development.

I also pray to St Anthony for help in finding things that I've lost. I've always done that, and it works! Psychologically, if you ask for outside help you stop trying so hard, and it takes some of the anxiety away – then the memory kicks in again. I firmly believe in prayer, and I feel that my work is a form of prayer. I ask for help on behalf of somebody else and the help comes through. My work is about helping people to be free from whatever is troubling them. I'm not actually moving people forward (they have to do that themselves), but I am clearing the patterns that hold them back. I feel as if I'm giving them an MOT. I look into the situation of the person who has the problem, their home and whoever is living with them – partner, mother, children, and, if I feel drawn to look more deeply at what's going on, there are often other issues needing attention. There's the fabric and history of the house, the location, the internal tensions, traumas from the past. This is such a big healing. Afterwards a person should be walking on air!

Usually, for me, the evening is not a good time to work on this level; for one thing I'm tired, yet ironically, I can't sleep afterwards! I need to feel in good form.

Although I am channelling, I am still using immeasurable energy. One clearing or healing a day is as much as I can and want to do. I could never sit down and do two. Carrying out a healing can be very beneficial to oneself too – if you are healing someone who has, for example, emotional problems – but when I'm dealing with Spirits, it needs a much stronger and different kind of energy.

MYSTERIOUS HAPPENINGS

SOME CASES stay in my mind, they're so unusual. There was one girl, living abroad, who was very unhappy in her marriage and very frustrated. She became very worked up, hysterical almost, about her partner, and ended up in a bad state because all sorts of mysterious goings-on were taking place in her home. During the course of the evening she would find unaccountable things happening – for example, the bath taps running when nobody had turned them on; children's electronic toys starting up on their own; lights switching themselves on. She had to do a lot of checking and double-checking before she was sure it wasn't someone playing tricks. Only then did she ask me to help.

Working with just her name and address and my pendulum, I detected an energy had really built up in the house because of pent-up feelings which were leading to destructive arguments. There were Spirits in the house as well, which I cleared. When things are really bad with a client I give them symbols to put in place, warding off evil. (These symbols are identical to the ones I use to swing my pendulum over when I am healing and clearing.) This lady put one of the symbols (which I had sent her as a form of protection) on her dressing table, facing towards the bed. When she woke up in the morning it had reversed itself. It had completely turned over so that it failed to have any effect! It was one of the symbols

I use against evil – and you can read into that incident what you will!

The electronic toy problem ceased and the bath taps stopped being turned on. I advised my client to place a lighted candle in the bedroom at night, and also a crystal, because it seemed to be at night when she was in bed that she felt vulnerable to some kind of psychic attack. She bought a bracelet made of crystals the next day and put it on her wrist. When she arrived home she found scratch marks right the way up her arm – the arm on which she was wearing the bracelet – similar to fingernail scratches. They could not possibly have been caused by the bracelet!

So I had to try and clear whatever had caused this. The client was also producing very powerful energy between herself and her partner. They were building up really negative energy and as fast as it was being cleared it was being reproduced. One morning she woke up and found scratch marks on her chest and around her throat – very distressing. She was sleeping alone, so there was no obvious explanation.

Things settled down again. My client was in her twenties, and she and her partner had created an unusual situation. What it actually shows is that you can help people to a certain extent. You can deal with Spirits, if Spirits are the problem. But when human nature intervenes and will not let that atmosphere settle down, then this unpleasantness manifests again. When her relationship settled down, everything else settled down.

Another client had a problem. She began to feel uncomfortable and rather distressed at night in her bedroom, she started to hear tapping on the window. I know the location of her room and there are no trees outside, nothing that could physically cause this noise. At the same time, several miles away in his own flat, her partner had also heard this tapping on his bedroom window. Their relationship was going through difficulties at the time. I cleared the energy and sent them both symbols to put up – and the tapping stopped! It had continued for about a week before I did the healing.

When I first started doing this work my psychic energy (for want of a better phrase) was not controlled properly and electrical equipment in particular started to malfunction. If I gave somebody one of my protective symbols to place in the home, often near the electric meter, I used to find they'd ring the next day and say that some electrical equipment in the home had stopped functioning. And in one case all the lights went out and they had to get in an electrician. I can only assume I hadn't trained the energy. Because I was new to this work I was channelling excessive amounts of energy to deal with problems that obviously needed far less. It was very embarrassing because I would take on someone's problem and really think I had cleared it. Then I'd get a call from the client saying they'd had to buy a new fridge!

PROCEDURES

MY APPROACH to this work is quite logical and scientific. When dowsing to find out the strength of the energy I'm dealing with I work on a scale of one to ten. I set my own numeric scale to detect the seriousness of any geopathic stress and/or discarnate energy.

Infrequently there can be a Curse placed on a place or a person that requires a slightly different approach. If, when dowsing for displaced discarnates, the answer is *yes*, I ask how many. Then I want to know how long they've been there – more than five years, more than ten, etc. Then I want to know what kind of energy it is. There are different groups of Spirit energies, and I have a chart that shows the kind of energies one might encounter, and this list includes a Curse. We have frequent interferences from discarnates in the aura, for example, right through to demonic forces, thankfully less common.

The darker the forces, the more effect they have on people. I ask, through my Higher Self, what intensity the force conveys using a gradient between one and ten, getting to know how strong their resistance will be. It's not just the type of energy, but the strength it conveys. I've been informed that there is a normal vibrational energy (similar in theory to a normal body temperature) for a human being and I've been given the figure of 2,100 vibrations (per second, I think). So we are all oscillating. If somebody is out of sorts their vibration goes down a little. If it's really low – say 1,900 –

they're either very ill and/or incredibly open to discarnates, because they're at such a low ebb. I always try to check people's vibrations before and after the healing. One can also measure the person's life force (which shows how affected they are by negative energy, also illness) and take a reading between one and ten. This is very helpful, especially if you measure again after the healing.

When a client first contacts me I take their name and address. It's all I need to know. I usually politely ask them not to give me more than the very basic facts, because I need to have a clear mind in order to get accurate information through the pendulum. What a client thinks is wrong is not necessarily the actual problem. So, through the *yes* and *no* workings of my pendulum, I first of all ask of my Higher Self if it is appropriate for me to do this particular work. It *could* be that I should not interfere. However, if *yes*, I ask if there's any geopathic stress. If so I'll ask what kind of stress. Maybe underground water, some form of escaping electricity which can cause problems, anything external like radar or power lines and boxes where electrical controls are housed. What you have to remember is that as individuals we all react differently to our environment. If there's a flu virus going around some people will get it and some people won't. You can't say categorically that everyone's going to be affected. But where problems of health and disquiet exist you have to investigate all areas of potential stress, like water or electrical rays, because they can be responsible for health and emotional problems. So that's why I check everything on the outside, as well as spiritual influences.

Geopathic stress is stress caused by our environment. The word comes from 'geo' meaning 'of the earth' and incorporates what is coming out through the ground or through the atmosphere and into our home. I usually swing the pendulum over an appropriate symbol, and ask that the place and its occupants be cleared of electrical or water rays, or whatever is indicated. Then I leave small symbols to be placed in the trouble spots inside the house. If I have successfully carried out this healing and clearing and the client's vibration is right up to 2,100 again, that is wonderful. It's a very good guideline.

I then have to turn my attention to any spiritual entities, if indeed they are present. Very often the 'polluted' atmosphere attracts discarnates, particularly water rays from underground 'black streams' – stagnant water well below the foundations of the property. Then I ask the Higher Self to send the discarnates to the Light or to their right and proper place. The pendulum spins round and round over the appropriate symbol until its job is done. Sometimes I ask the Spirit if it wants to go. I do these things intuitively. And then I ask if it's gone – *yes* or *no*? I ask if there are any discarnates left – I might have removed some and not others, so I check. Then I create a shield of white light around the client using my particular symbol – the Peace symbol.

But because I'm interested to learn *why* the person is having this experience – as is the client – I like to look at the surrounding history. Apart from finding out how long the Spirit has been around, I can then often, psychically or clairvoyantly, find out if there's a personal scenario, which I follow through using the pendulum. So, for example, if I sense that there could be an old woman connected with this Spirit I can go on to find out what the history is around her that might have had a connection with the house, for example. There might be no connection at all, but whatever negativity there was around that Spirit in human form, the Spirit will be attracted to something of that in the person they are worrying. Therefore there is this attraction of Spirits to people who have their own problems. I always find this aspect very interesting.

You can build up a very good picture, at times, of past lives. Some people use regression in order to find out if they've had other lives; not everybody believes in this theory. I think I'm sitting on the fence over this one, but I have to acknowledge that I sometimes intuitively pick up on a strong 'storyline', and this scenario seems to be connected with the use of some form of regression or some kind of hypnotherapy or psychotherapy. I think that the past lives that I go along with are probably bloodlines, in other words something that occurred way down genetically in a person's bloodline even if it dates back hundreds of years – male or female. I think there can be a genetic memory, and in some people, 'past life' experiences come back to haunt them. The latest theory by experts working with DNA is called Epigenetics, the idea that our genes have a 'memory', that the lives of our grandparents – from the air they breathed to the food they ate, even the things they saw – can directly affect us, decades later. A major shift from conventional thinking – but one that dovetails very neatly into my work, shared, of course, by many others.

I tend to subscribe to the genetics theory, although there *have* been staggering examples of verifiable memories of past lives, particularly from children. I'm not certain we come back to learn different lessons or to perfect different lives. There might be only one life, or many, but I can't be sure. I feel that the *present* one is the *only* one that matters and I don't have much inclination to look and see what happened before this life. Very often people feel that such-and-such an experience has happened before, or else feel they must be learning something in this 'incarnation'. Perhaps we try to convince ourselves of that because it makes us comfortable. It does create a certain amount of comfort to feel that we are in this life because we have come in to do whatever we choose to do this time around. I think I'm still of the Christian outlook where we come into the world and work to perfect ourselves in preparation for the next world. I feel more comfortable with that, but I have that opinion without any proof either way; I cannot and do not discard other philosophies. So many people do feel there are past lives, and that they have a responsibility in some way to make good or make amends, and many go through hypnotherapy and psychotherapy to research and investigate any other 'lives' they have had.

From my point of view, someone who remembers a past life may have had a Spirit possessing him during that life, or his death could have been a very bad experience. It could have been murder. He might have gone immediately to his death never having had a chance to prepare for passing on. We used to call it 'not being in a state of grace'. There might have been something around him at death that was very negative. Then if you go through a negative process by reliving the past and bring it back into the present, you might see what has happened. That is what regression is all about. A person relives circumstances around that moment in time, bringing up everything they can remember. Because they can't just pick and choose their memories they are also picking up the negative activities.

A lot of people I know in this line of work do not approve of regression, particularly if it's being done by so called 'spiritual' people who do it through their mediumship, or work on the spiritual level. It does constitute a danger, and not every sincere person is necessarily able to deal with subsequent problems. If it is done in a responsible and supervised way it may be all right, but many people are not responsible. I mean, we are dabbling in the unknown, aren't we – the *unknown* being the consequences of our actions!

It has now been proved that we can recall embryonic memories from before we were born, certain experiences in the womb. About thirty years ago one would have thought this was nonsense. But we know now that children can respond and remember things from the womb. We also know that our bodies are made up of around 70 per cent water –

and water retains memory. We are made up of genes which are passed down from two families to a child. So we've got this bodily/genetic capacity for memory. We've got all these genes that influence our entire make-up.

I do believe we bring loads of 'pre-recorded material' into the world with us. They say babies are pure. They are, in their hearts and minds, because they have had no experience, but not regarding the genes they bring with them — when you look at their hands (as I have as a palmist) it's already laid out what sort of person they are likely to be. So although they are innocent at the moment they are born, how they're going to turn out is already weighted in favour of their genetic inheritance.

I like to simplify everything, and know that when I give readings to people, or use some psychometry, they are very happy and reassured to see me using a 'tool', something as an outward form of guidance, and some clients are never as convinced, sitting with a clairvoyant, as to where the information is coming from. They wonder if it's merely imagination! If I can show them a tarot card, for example, then they are happy. So I believe that's how I appear to authenticate any healing or clearing I am carrying out — it appears that the pendulum is doing the work… but it is simply my 'tool'!

RESCUING THE LIVING

I DON'T think all people are suited to working in the same way as myself, although my students do love to learn this clearing process. I don't even like the word 'clearing', but it does seem to describe a form of cleansing, making space to improve one's life without unnatural hindrance. Rescue work is a widely used expression, coming probably from the Spiritualist Church. They're rescuing souls. However, I seem to be in demand, almost totally, for rescuing *people* from *harmful* energies. I'm sending these discarnate energies to their rightful place, wherever that is, so often I'm actually rescuing the living!

Where there are no harmful issues, these Spirits are just waiting to be sent on their way. But they're not all good. Rescue sounds as if something is in distress and wants to go. Sometimes that is the case and sometimes it isn't. Just as people are good and bad, so Spirits are good and bad as well. If somebody has been born pure like every other baby and if during the course of their life has turned to evil ways and not given a single thought to the good of their soul, they haven't done the job they were sent here to do, which was actually to look after their own spiritual welfare and prepare themselves in some way. They haven't done their stuff. When they die I believe their soul belongs to God. Their Spirit is the disembodied part of them which may be attached to their earthly life. If they have lived good lives, it's possible (I suppose) that they may stay here to help people. But they might be quite destructive – like poltergeists, for example. I couldn't myself use the term 'rescue work' for a poltergeist. It's more a case of clearing it and sending it to the where it needs to go.

I believe we are part of God. The Spirit is just the disembodiment of that particle which is a human being. It can be an unhappy Spirit or happy Spirit. Of course, many people don't believe in the soul, but I believe that if we are a fragment of something really enormous – our Creator – then that little bit is the soul, which has inhabited our body while we have been alive.

It is possible to clear an atmosphere, or person, or house, and then have that space sullied again by the person himself still living a certain harmful way of life that is their *choice* – i.e. drinking too much, being unkind, abusive or living to excess. There are people who are really full of hate or such like; they've got strong emotions that burn them up. Prejudices can be very powerful. And some people dislike themselves, that's quite common; and then you get problems like eating disorders, attempted suicides, depression, a hate of life sometimes – 'Can't bear it; don't want to live another day!' These feelings can be very much *enhanced* by evil Spirits.

An illness can affect somebody for years so that it almost becomes a way of life, and even if you clear the discarnates away, if that person's outlook has become very negative (not just with their own illness but the whole concept of their body and other people's bodies not being OK) then other discarnates might find a way in later on. There's insanity, which is an obvious one really; jealousy; low self-esteem; negativity – that's a very broad one but some people can be so negative that they are opening themselves up to 'invasion', as I call it. Rejection (of something or someone) or a feeling of having been rejected, is a problem that goes very deep in the human psyche. Either you do the rejecting or are being rejected. If you've got an issue about rejection all the time, it's so negative it casts a shadow over your life. There's also self-centredness and self-destruction. There is a lot of self, self, self here. Self-punishment, and selfishness, manifest in human lives frequently. Self-limitation is an outlook you might not think of as a major personality problem, but by limiting yourself you're closing all the doors. You are limiting yourself to saying, 'I never need a holiday – I'm fine with my boring work, my unhappy marriage' or 'I *can't* do it': that's limiting yourself, leaving yourself open to all kinds of negativity.

The bad side of sexuality is here – abuse, perversion, promiscuity; these are all things that are very negative and damaging to somebody. There's also spiritual suicide (I had to think about that one when I was looking at it). In other words, you're almost falling on your own sword – you don't want to own up to the spiritual side of yourself, and so you want to destroy it and that's quite common if you think deeply enough. If somebody doesn't want to know the spiritual side of this world and completely cuts it off, then they're denying another dimension. They're denying that there is something outside themselves, perhaps life after death. All the things that give us a little bit of hope. Realistic, you may say, but it can be very negative too. And then there is having an unforgiving nature – a trait hard to break.

These are very big issues touching many of us. Some are just aspects of ourselves. But they all indicate that if one of these negative aspects appears to be the dominant energy, then the Spirit attaching itself to that person will make things ten times worse. Such is the strength of these harmful energies.

Very simply that's how it is – addiction, child abuse, depression are all part of this. Depression is one of the worst things; every line of defence closes down. Another negative state is escapism: one has to think about that sometimes. It's actually not owning up to the reality of a situation. So if you are not looking at things straight and objectively, you can be very vulnerable. You might not be doing anything wrong but you haven't got your feet on the ground. So you're not grounded in reality – that can make life very difficult.

Over and over again, when I've dowsed for these characteristics (usually without a client knowing) and I've mentioned two or three of these traits that have come up, they can relate to them. They're either experiencing these difficulties in themselves or those around them.

I have to be accurate when dowsing for these issues. But the right thing always comes up. This Programme of negative states is very interesting. There's hardly anything there that you can't interpret as being a driving negative force. But when a discarnate is pushing you in this direction you are very vulnerable. Being vulnerable doesn't mean being negative, but if there is no strong belief system or faith in anything – almost like the fool card in the tarot – you are tripping along and can't see what's in front of you. Then these influences can knock you sideways and you can get attacked psychically.

Going back to what I was relating when I went back to my flat in the Docklands in 1991, and the poltergeist experience. I myself was in a vulnerable state. I don't think there were any of these issues, but I was upset because my flat hadn't been looked after properly. I wasn't ranting and raving, but nevertheless I must have created a negative atmosphere which made it quite easy for what was already in the flat to start doing its work. I played a part in that. I do recognise that now. If I had moved back, been determined not to be affected by the neglect and not over-reacted, simply dealt with it then, I wouldn't have had that psychic attack.

We can attract negative energies if we go to visit somebody in hospital, or go to a funeral or mental institution. We should really clear ourselves in some way. In the Catholic tradition, people cross themselves as a form of protection. Just that gesture of crossing ourselves is enough. Not everybody goes around crossing themselves, but that is a gesture of asking God to please take care of us. You can ask a higher power to protect you – but please don't turn to superstitious practices.

A Programme can go on and on unless somebody comes to the rescue of that Spirit and turns it around. Love of alcohol may be someone's problem, but it shouldn't rule the person's whole life. We all have to have a balance sheet. Addiction is terrible. It is an illness. If we go down that path and have given in to every negative pressure that comes along and have not been a strong person in any way, there's quite a lot of 'clearing' to do. But if someone has been a good person, has inherited an addiction and has lost the battle, then it really isn't such a difficult job to help them.

My work is very varied. I have a lovely client who comes to me, and has done so regularly for ten years since he realised that I could dowse an area to pick up positive and negative conditions in a house. He rents, and moves frequently. He is very sensitive and picks up every little psychic thing. It started when he had a reading and was going to move. He had to choose one of three flats – 47, 59 or 53 – and I dowsed to see which one, if any, pointed to being the right one for him. He wanted to know if I could pick up anything particularly good or bad. Since then he has appeared regularly. I use the dowsing to see if his prospective flat is fine. He is an intelligent man and there is just this side to him that completely and utterly trusts the dowsing. Sometimes we go through the procedure on the phone. He's moved about eight times in the last ten years – not, I hasten to add, because something isn't right, but his lease will run out or there's a fire in the basement, etc.

There are many light sides to this work. The clearings I

tend to illustrate in this book are the more dramatic ones. I've got several cards on a friend who is really terribly sensitive. He had a flatmate who was really into spiritualism and training to be a medium. He felt, as I did, that she was bringing some problematic influences into the flat. Not terrible things, but just enough to make him feel uncomfortable. She was a depressive and on medication, and really shouldn't have been getting into this work, which she had to stop eventually because it was getting the better of her. But all the while she was bringing in these Spirits, my poor friend was having these 'visitations' during the night because he is so easily affected by these things. A big price to pay for innocently taking on a flatmate!

HAUNTINGS

THE VARIOUS homes I have lived in have mostly had problems, many personal to me. At my first home when I was a child I used to see a sea of faces coming in and out of my consciousness when I lay in bed at night. Looking back, I think this was happening to me because I was rather vulnerable as a child. Although I had parents who loved and cared for me, it's possible that I picked up an undercurrent of emotional difficulties that were not out in the open – difficulties that I now, as an adult, understand. So I've got the feeling these psychic experiences were related in some measure to circumstances reigning in the home.

When married, we moved a couple of times and everything was fine. Then, with three children, we moved to a large house in Sussex. The property consisted of two semi-detached farm cottages and a series of farm buildings. At one end was an old dairy and a huge tiled room where they used to hang game. It had belonged to the bailiff of a large estate. We renovated it and converted it into one big house.

My youngest daughter Julia's bedroom was in the part of the property that had been one of the semi-detached cottages. She used to see the ghost of an old lady walk through her bedroom, through one door, across the room and pass into the next room. I didn't know what to make of it. After we converted the cottages my daughter Linda, whose room was right at the other end of the property, told me the old lady had come into her room too!

We turned the game larder into a games room for table tennis and darts for the teenagers. Once when my husband John, and I were out, my mother-in-law was staying there keeping an eye on the children when Linda said she saw a man go through to the games room. My mother-in-law was very worried because the house was isolated, and she phoned the police. They came out and scoured the whole area. But when Linda described this man to me, it was obviously a ghost. He had a long, flowing coat. And it was spooky in the games room! I never liked going down there on my own at night. I never saw anything but I believed the children were telling the truth. I could feel the atmosphere, and I didn't really like that part of the property.

We eventually changed it from a games room into a beautiful living room. We put in windows and doors and removed all the glazed tiles, which seemed to cleanse it. Moving the fabric that had been holding on to something for years and years shifted the atmosphere. It had been almost entirely tiled because they didn't have refrigeration in the original era and it had to be as cold as possible. Animals had been butchered there and I think this energy was trapped. We removed a ceiling and exposed the rafters – who knows what we let out!

If I had been able to look at the place with the skills I have now I would have been able to find out more. As a mother I did have to pretend that I didn't mind going down into the room. This kind of atmosphere can be created by something that's happened in a place or because of the people who've lived there. It can be so many different things. It could have been built over an old burial ground, as it was next to a church (part of the original estate). We lived there for eleven years and during the renovations I think we got rid of all the negative energy and it was both physically and spiritually cleansed. Apparently orphans were housed there and looked after by nuns during World War II – another piece of the jigsaw.

I had no more problems until as a single person I moved to a basement flat in Hove. It was not haunted, but after a year or two my energy levels dropped. Anyway, as I have said, my good friend Jim Ives cleared the problem, which was connected with electrical 'rays'. I was a little suspicious of his methods at first, especially as he used to dowse over symbols. I have to be very careful now when I suggest using this method because people might associate it with magic! Despite my concern I felt much better in myself and the process was a real inspiration, and my entry into the work I do now.

I have learnt through experience that my vulnerability to Spirits or atmosphere was sometimes because I was at a low ebb; my consequent negativity was causing things to happen around me, but sometimes it was caused by problems in the house itself. Therefore I'm very conscious of this when I'm looking in to other people's problems. You've really got to distinguish straight away who and what you are dealing with, because you can't clear the energy unless you know exactly what it is – the environment, the client or a mixture of both. If people are emotionally unstable they can stir things up in an atmosphere like dust in a room.

One lady who was recommended to me said she would really like me to go to her home. I only visit clients on rare occasions but I decided she needed some support. It was an old house and had a graveyard nearby – which was the first thing I noticed. Old electrical cables were running into the house from masts. I dowsed first for geopathic stress and the thing that came out most strongly were water rays. My investigations showed stagnant water under the property. This is called black water because it is not running freely. It tends to build up under the foundations of a property, and historically attracts earthbound Spirits. I also found electrical rays. I went into a cupboard under the stairs and it was quite clear that there was some strong seepage of electricity there (reminiscent of my own problem years previously). I put symbols over the meter to try to keep the leakage in check, and I advised her to have the electrical circuit looked at.

When symbols are placed over the meter they deflect the electricity rays and also deflect the water rays as well. It may sound strange but this energy from water and electricity seems to run round the electrical circuit. The only proof I have is that it works! The way to deflect these rays is to put a very powerful symbol with the blank side up, so that the pattern cannot be seen, and it deflects the negativity instead of absorbing it. That's as much as you can do in those circumstances. Most times it works, and if it doesn't there's not much else you can do about geopathic stress.

There were some discarnates in the house I visited, not connected to the owner or her partner. Her vibrations (I dowsed for these) were good and everybody who lived there was fine. At no time did my client say they were affected by this negative energy, just aware of it. So they were strong in themselves. I cleared the discarnates.

The large attic had bad energy and was over the client's bedroom. She used to hear footsteps above. There was also a playhouse at the bottom of the garden. As I went around the house into different rooms, I didn't need my pendulum. I could feel, as I walked from room to room, the various energies. The kitchen-diner felt fine. But other rooms had a lot of bad energy, and I investigated this while she was there with me to try and find out what sort of discarnates they were.

When I consulted my chart there seemed to be a kind of Imprint on the rooms themselves of whatever had been happening there in previous years. The rooms were almost speaking to me. I picked up that there had been some kind of child abuse there, physical but not sexual. The discarnates were not the problem initially, but were there because of the unhealthy, unhappy atmosphere. The general atmosphere needed cleansing. Certain places, like the playhouse, had really bad energy trapped there, and I think something horrible had happened – perhaps a child had been locked in. I felt that this had happened in the house as well as the playhouse. Children had been crying and adults shouting. It was a most unpleasant atmosphere. When I left I really hoped I had cleared it.

In a day or so the client said that the footsteps in the attic had stopped and she felt much calmer. In the same way that flies are attracted to a piece of bad meat, the discarnates at this property had some kind of need to be there. They weren't necessarily bad or doing anything harmful, but were there because the atmosphere was tainted. Once this is cleared they won't come back.

The footsteps were a hangover of the Imprint from the violent scenes that had taken place, and my client was very psychic. Make no bones about it, if you are living in a house containing these sort of energies, you are going to be aware of them. They are unwelcome guests, however benign. The nearness of the graveyard was also an influence. Around graveyards there are a lot of Spirits of people who haven't made a quick passage to their next place of rest. And you can always feel the floating population, because that is what they are.

I've done one large-scale clearing in France which was a residue of a battle in World War II. Canadian soldiers landed on 19 August 1942 at Pourville, near Dieppe, and were met with a tirade of gunfire. It was a massacre, and hundreds died on the beach. A friend who lived there said she always had a sense that there was a cloud over the place, and there were also a series of nasty accidents near the seafront on the main road. A child was fatally injured when a motorist accidentally went into reverse and shot out of his garage on to the pavement. Another child was killed by a motorcyclist after leaving the beach.

I visited the resort and certainly felt there was a real heaviness in certain areas, especially in one of the lanes near the beach that was overhung with trees. There seemed to be a whole residue of souls and Spirits in the atmosphere along with the terrible sense of mass death that had been left behind. When I returned home I dowsed a postcard of Pourville. As I cleared the atmosphere I felt as if the sun was shining brightly over the entire area. I felt extraordinarily fulfilled. It was a totally different feeling for me, a different kind of clearance because I wasn't weeding out people's problems. I was dealing with tragic death on a vast scale as far as I could. It's extraordinary how something like that can be so effective using only a pendulum and a symbol. But I suppose that with spiritually, just as there's really no such thing as time, there is no such thing as size or area. So there is no reason why any area, big or small, can't be dealt with in this way. I asked for all the unhappiness to go and for all the Spirits and the energy that was pervading the place to be released. In this case I did feel that 'rescue work' was exactly what I thought I was doing because those soldiers had done nothing wrong. I think you get little tunnels of energy sometimes, as you do with extreme weather, and I think this was probably causing the accidents to occur in the area. It was a sort of re-enactment of collisions of vehicles and tanks, and unnecessary death.

It was a place where you could very easily clairvoyantly capture the scene. I think that from the moment the soldiers started to come up the beach, tanks and aircraft were gunning them down. The Allies landed in a very ill-considered way. They were thrown in at the deep end. The hope was that if 1,000 soldiers landed and 200 survived they might be able to get through. This was horrific. It was even worse in World War I. Thanks goodness I haven't had to do any clearings connected with that war. I don't think I could bear it.

Clearing concentration camps has been dealt with by others. There are many people involved in this work. Some camps have been turned into gardens of remembrance and meditation. I don't think that would be possible if you still had bad atmospheres.

Some of the cases I have been involved in have made me cringe. Some people feel that really difficult energies should actually be left alone rather than delved into and dug up. There's always the other way of looking at it – that you should leave all this and not disturb it. But I really think if there's any energy that can be cleared it's like opening all the windows in the morning and letting stale air out and fresh air in.

One client contacted me some time after I had cleared her house. She wanted to have counselling. She was having a very difficult time with her husband. I realised she was an innocent bystander to the energy that was being put out and kept going by her husband, who was a very problematic personality. There was no longer anything wrong with the house. His negativity had created an energy of its own and there were certainly Spirits around. She was an artist and very sensitive.

He was actually creating this, so I had to clear these energies as well as I could. I did manage to clear a good bit of the house, but funnily enough I wasn't able to clear all of it. There was still an area upstairs that caused a problem. I think his influence was so strong that whatever energy I cleared would be replaced the next day. That's how it is if somebody is very difficult or depressed. You are trying to clear something that's being replenished all the time. But my 'best' was good enough for this lady and she was extremely grateful. It gave her a clear space again and she felt better and was able to reinstate herself as a person. Before, she had been feeling tremendously under the influence of her husband. She no longer felt oppressed.

I picked up seven Spirits there and gave her a protective symbol for every room. There were also water rays beneath the house. The husband had what I call an 'off the scale' reading, very high, and was under a Programme of Revenge and Bitterness. He was influenced by a particular discarnate that I felt had been there from his conception. Although I removed that, I felt he'd got such an inbuilt Programme that I think it would have needed a long process of work to really change him. I wasn't asked to do any more and I didn't offer. I was more interested in my client regaining her own power, which in itself was a remarkable achievement.

On another occasion she asked me to help a friend whose husband had become obsessed with his therapist! He was having electrical therapy for a limb over which he had no muscle control. He became hateful to his wife. He was seeking attention from his therapist, was absolutely obsessed with her, and couldn't at the present time stand his wife near him although they had been reasonably happily married for about forty years.

In the home there were three discarnates, all from past lives. He had a personality Programme of Resentment, Complaining, Fear and Sexual Promiscuity. There were bad Spirits in the home encouraging his behaviour. His wife was free of Spirits but her vibration was very low at 1,500 (it should be 2,100). She was totally worn out, so they were both suffering, each in their own way. She in turn had a Programme of Jealousy, Complaining and Despair. She was programmed to respond to this bad relationship. He was turning to somebody else and she was jealous. He was resentful of his condition. She felt rejected and desperate because of his promiscuity. An ill-fated pair, if ever I saw one.

I studied the therapist and found through dowsing that, although she was unprofessional, she wasn't necessarily encouraging him. It was all about the husband and wife's problems. She was unprofessional possibly in that she was too friendly, but that was as far as it went. The electrical treatment was largely to blame. The man saw his wife as not being helpful and was very resentful; the therapist was very helpful. There was a real fear in him that his complaint would worsen. I picked up all that although I knew nothing about them, only the name and address, which is the only information I ever require. I very seldom meet my clients, and they are usually referred to me by others.

I reported back to my original client and she confirmed all my findings. I cleared all the Spirits and I also gave the client distance healing. I have heard things are better between them although the condition of his leg muscles has not improved. But this is a physical problem and not something I set out to deal with.

A CURSE

I WAS contacted by a man who already had a good knowledge of psychic matters. He worked in the media and was very articulate. He felt he'd had nothing but bad luck, although he appeared to be very successful. There was a negativity which seemed to have affected the male line of his family. His wife had left him and his father had had the same experience. People walked out of this man's life, or fell out with him, in a rather melodramatic way.

I spent a long time working on his case and I uncovered more than I had ever done with anyone else. I had been given a list of people's soul levels – a well-known chart in spiritual circles. When we come into the world we have potential in many ways, which I believe can be seen through the palms of the hand and an astrological chart, but there is nothing documented about our spiritual potential. We do have access to a scale of soul levels – these include Guide, Guardian Angel, Angel of Light and Master. I dowse over this chart when I'm dealing with somebody over the phone who has a somewhat abstract problem. It helps me to gauge where a person is coming from spiritually. I decided to find this man's level because he seemed to have very deep understanding. I found that spiritually he came under the level of Guide and, interestingly, he always wanted to sort out the family and help people along.

It became obvious to me that there was a very deep problem connected with him and his family before him.

A CURSE

I knew that he was having what he thought was bad luck, and he felt it had been handed down in some way. He had a normal vibration, so it wasn't actually affecting his equilibrium or his health, but he did have a discarnate with him from a past life and with a very strong influence. This was something he had inherited; that's the only way I can describe it. He'd brought this Spirit into the present life at about the age of twelve. He had used a Ouija board around about that time and I think that's when it started to manifest. He had also been professionally regressed because he wanted to see if there was anything from a past life influencing him. This Spirit was a bit like a virus that was being passed on from one incarnation to the next.

So I studied his Programme and came up with Restlessness, Self-destruction, Murder, Jealousy, Adultery and Depression. This discarnate was bringing these characteristics in. Then I asked, through the pendulum, what this very strong Spirit he was carrying was, and I was told it was a Curse. Well, that really sparked the investigation.

He had had the strangest things happen to him. His wife had left him for no apparent reason, had gone to live in another country and stopped communicating with him, and he felt totally mystified. Then his daughter had joined her and stopped communicating too. The same thing had happened to his father. His mother had left without any kind of notice and without any obvious problems in the marriage. His son had brought a girlfriend home and after going out with him for several months, she cut him in the street and never spoke to him again. There was something going through the male line; he was right. Women would cut him out of their lives without any reason whatsoever. His latest girlfriend had sat down to dinner with him and his son. Suddenly she'd said she had to go and called a taxi, never to return. There was something very strange going on, and every time this happened he was terribly upset.

A CURSE

After I gave healing to this man I had the experience of soft voices coming out of my telephone, which was a very disconcerting experience. Undoubtedly I'd aroused something somewhere because the telephone is a conduit. I could not pick up what they were saying. I could hear the rise and fall of a man's voice and a woman — it was just at the pitch where, if I'd have had some kind of magnification, I'd have been able to hear it. I taped it and also left it on my machine for a long time for other people to hear. The phone would ring, the answering machine would switch on automatically and these voices could be heard. It happened several times while I was dealing with this client. I knew I was picking up something that had stirred a reaction in the other world. Also, whenever I gave him distant healings, this man had to go to bed and sleep for a few hours. Each time there was a huge clearing going on which was affecting him physically. He told me that on one occasion he was talking to somebody at the time of the healing and he just couldn't keep his eyes open.

A month later, the discarnate was still around him. Things were gradually getting better after the second clearing, although he was very exhausted. He promised to ring me in a week. I started looking to see where this Curse had come from. I found that it went right back to a point in history where the Incas were invaded by the Spanish, and on one occasion they had attacked tribes during a festival when they were off guard. I discovered that a Spanish soldier had lured a girl away from the village. He had been sexually involved with her and made her feel important — she had given him information which he had acted on, and was therefore partly responsible for the attack. When the girl realised what had happened and that he had been using her, she screamed a Curse at him and every male in his line, because he had been disloyal to her and let her down. It must have been a very powerful Curse. As it turned out, my client was of Spanish descent. Whether the Curse had gone on and on, passed down through the generations, or whether it had come out into the open when he used the Ouija board, I'm not certain.

I picked up psychically that he needed to ask for forgiveness. I couldn't remove the Curse on my own. I knew he and his son had to do something. He collected crystals; his house was absolutely full of them. Crystals have very strong vibrations and he spent a lot of time with them in his study. I felt that such magnified energy was not helping him, and told him to get rid of two thirds of the crystals or not to display them together. He took my advice. The energy was too strong, and one has to discriminate against 'too much of a good thing'. He had to build up his own resistance, so that when the Curse was finally cleared, he would be able to protect himself in the future.

A few days later he phoned me and told me that he and his son had gone down to the beach. They had each taken a crystal and had thrown them into the sea as a gesture to their ancestor's wrongdoing. They said that they were sorry for anything their ancestors had done. They both cried and cried. Afterwards he felt there was a softening of the hold of the discarnate, and he felt distinctly freer. I said I would pray with him for forgiveness, and use the words *enough is enough*. I prayed that God would be merciful to him. This was a very powerful and unusual case.

One man could never hold on his conscience what those Spanish soldiers had done, but this man and his son had both tried to get across how sorry they were. He'd been living for years with that bad luck, and it always seemed to be somebody else's fault. If you had gone back to the original Curse, that soldier might have felt it wasn't his fault either and that he was only doing his job.

I never met this man, but I felt as if I knew him intimately because we spent hours and hours on the telephone. A lot of counselling was done, side by side with the spiritual cleansing, and I am so grateful that I was able to handle this case.

THE DOMINATRIX

ONE OF my clients was a call girl, a dominatrix. She had loaned money to somebody who she thought was a friend, then couldn't get it back. She and a friend had concocted a spell (a dangerous practice to get involved in) to encourage this person to return the money, but it had backfired on her. It wasn't a spell to cast him into eternal damnation or anything like that, but she said that afterwards he was more against giving the money back to her than ever!

I found a discarnate with her, one of the really strong ones that could be called a demonic force. This showed powerful energy being used for the worst cause – it had been around her for nearly two years at a very high intensity. I didn't know at this stage what she did for a living, but I found she had a very interesting Programme when I dowsed. She was operating on Sadism, Self-punishment, Sexual Promiscuity, Despair and Cruelty. She had started off as a call girl, but a dominatrix is more highly paid and, quite honestly, somebody who does a job like this in many cases does get pleasure out of it. She'd probably moved into that Programme quite naturally, but hadn't always been like that. She was in her thirties.

She definitely had this force attached to her, and it was connected to her work. She didn't feel guilty about what she did, but she wasn't happy either. She had difficulty with certain personal relationships and with making close friends, and felt a lot of jealousy around her. So it wasn't surprising that because she had this pretty nasty energy around, the magic wasn't working properly.

I cleared her twice, and the second time that particular energy left. Something much milder remained in her aura. She wasn't clear. There was a little something that wasn't completely right spiritually. Her problem was that she was much too open (meaning unprotected) and she was on a rather seedy side of life as far as her job was concerned. The indication was that she was the sort of person who unless she really changed her way of life – interestingly she did have quite a strong spiritual side – was likely to pick up a harmful energy again. When you're beating the life out of somebody for money I can't think you'd be very sensitive to what's around you, and maybe she didn't realise how hugely significant this energy was. She was too open and didn't stop to think that this way of life could be harmful to her. I think when women go into prostitution they have several options available to them. They can simply lie back and think of England (!) or they can be asked to perform different services – and that's where personal choices lie. She was somebody who was open to Spirits, and anything anyone suggested as well. At the end of the day you've got to be pretty tough to do that work.

Quite a few prostitutes have come to me for readings over the years. They have personal problems like everybody else. They're perfectly normal – they breathe, sleep and eat and have love lives like everybody else. Mostly, prostitution takes a person down a pathway where they are not meeting really spiritual people, so they are not feeding or nurturing that part of their nature. It's not about sex. It's about money.

Something in a client's hand might indicate that they are fairly highly sexed and are also content to make easy money. Very often prostitutes have a lucky streak. They have a prominent sun line in their palm, which means they can stand out in a crowd. Factors like this might give me a clue what clients do for a living. But prostitution is not something you can pinpoint as easily as being a librarian or a writer. Mostly people do have other talents and they're simply doing this work to make money to finance themselves. But it's dangerous.

AUTOMATIC WRITING

HER VIBRATION was down to 1,900. She was an attractive, intelligent woman with a charming personality. She came to me for a reading and happened to tell me there was something 'not right' where she was working. When I investigated with the pendulum using my question and answer technique, I found she was being affected by negative energy. Electricity was filtering in from cables and pylons outside the building. I cleared that electricity out of her body and brought her vibration back to the correct level. I looked to see if there was anything else in the large, old house where she lived. Well, there were five discarnates – four were really detrimental to her health and state of mind, the other was just present.

She needed more exercise and more positive thought to give herself an opportunity to form more intimate relationships. She needed a nudge to make her life fulfilling.

This dark energy had existed in the building for thirty years. Many developmental courses had been held there and mediums had also been trained. This woman was good at her job but she wasn't making the same efforts in her personal life. Her Programme was Restlessness, Ego – she was somebody who needed to shine – Depression, Excesses, Dislike of Women. She was having a terrific problem with relationships and that was highlighted. She was working with mediums and the courses she ran included automatic writing. I advised her to take a break from all this. It is possible to stir up a lot of negativity with automatic writing.

She was only forty but was very run down. Her adrenal glands were not functioning properly so her resistance was low and she felt something was around all the time.

She sought out the appropriate counselling and the situation began to improve. Some people just need clearing. Others need to grow up a bit and listen to themselves. I never force the idea of counselling on anybody, but if it follows on naturally after the 'clearing' there is always a great benefit.

SISTERS

ONE OF my clients was having a problem with her sister. There wasn't much difference in their ages but she felt her sister was trying to control everything and being very awkward.

My client was getting a real phobia about her sister. They were dealing with their dead mother's estate at the time and what was going on between them was developing into an exceptionally nasty situation. I checked the sister's house with the pendulum. There was no geopathic stress, but two discarnates had been in the house for three years. They were reflecting Conscious Control and this energy had attached itself to the sister. I also picked up Sexual Abuse, Abuse of Animals, Child Abuse and Anger. I think the sister had been abused as a child. She was desperately trying to control things now because she had felt out of control during childhood. After the healing her vibrations were normal. Everything completely changed. The sisters went out to lunch and had a really nice time!

Realistically, the sister had been traumatised by the death of her mother, who might have been a real support when she was a child, and losing this parent made her feel she was floundering. She was trying to have her own way, which is what people do when they feel a bit out of control. She was inviting in negative energy, which was encouraging her to be absolutely horrible. It did have a happy ending, though!

A MUSICIAN

A MUSICIAN once asked me to go round to his apartment. He was a composer and performer. His place was dreadfully untidy, and none too clean, and he looked as though he'd been dragged through a hedge backwards! This is not a criticism, simply a statement of fact, helping to set the scene. The *only* thing that really mattered to him was his music. There was absolutely nowhere to sit; it was real chaos. This terribly nice man came out of the wreckage and made me a cup of tea. He'd lived here for about seven years and felt there was something really wrong with the flat.

He was thirty-seven and very sensitive, as you would expect, but he just didn't look after himself at all. Everything I checked showed shortcomings. Fortunately there was no geopathic stress and he *could* have had a lovely home; it was on the top floor of an old house with gables. But he was a most unhappy and depressed man. First of all I looked at his chakras (an invisible energy system in our body). His liver and digestive system, and heart and lungs were in a poor condition. So I closed his chakras, which helped the organs to function better. I also balanced his aura and unblocked the crown chakra. You don't want this chakra wide open (making you too vulnerable spiritually) but neither do you want it blocked. He was capable of receiving higher thoughts but he seemed blocked and his vibrations were very low, 1,800. He was living on tea and coffee. He didn't eat any fruit or vegetables – his diet was appalling and he was using drugs.

A MUSICIAN

He was not a drug addict but he smoked pot, possibly used cocaine as well. He was lacking in everything nourishing, and needed constructive and spiritual support, recreation and fresh air. The latter are such obvious things to anybody, but he hadn't recognised them. He never walked. He never opened the windows. He had lost his love of life. Although there was no geopathic stress in his flat, negative rays were coming in via a satellite dish. The chemicals in his body were tantamount to being overwhelming, and he had precious little on the positive side to balance it out.

He had three discarnates in his aura which had been present for four years. He was very pasty, gaunt, thin and didn't move well at all. I also noticed that the brow chakra, which controls one's intelligence, was open. He wasn't questioning anything. He had been in a relationship, one which had felt important to him, but his lady had just drifted off, and he didn't really understand why. He had a Programme of Abandonment, Betrayal, Alcoholism, Ego and Failure. With a bit of a push from these discarnates he could easily have gone down the road to alcoholism. The abandonment certainly reflected how he was feeling. There was also a sense of betrayal and failure. He wasn't a failure as a musician but at that time he didn't feel that anything was going right for him. With this Programme he tended to rather dislike himself. He couldn't see he was an attractive person. He had guilt and low self-esteem. He carried the negative trait of Spiritual Suicide (which is a deliberate attempt to cut yourself off from the spiritual side of your nature) and he was trying to block out any finer feelings. But he did seek help from me!

This healing came in the nick of time. He really could have gone down a slippery slope. We really hit it off. I understood him.

I carried out another healing on him a month later. He was much better. He had a wonderfully equipped music room,

A MUSICIAN

and once he got in there and got his electronic music going he felt much better. He'd tidied up physically and spiritually.

Discarnates come into the aura when you are at a low ebb and not well. They stay in the aura until you meet a therapist, a medium or clairvoyant who can clear the aura. Sometimes if you go into deep meditation the aura will clear automatically.

GUILTY HORMONES

ONE CLIENT I treated had all her chakras blocked, which meant that hardly anything of a sensitive nature was getting through, but her soul level was high (I can observe this through my dowsing). This was a somewhat unusual situation. I unblocked the chakras and gave her a major healing. I also looked at her health. She was depressed and self-centred. There *could* have been an unwanted presence, but in her case there wasn't. She was forty-seven and menopausal, which probably made her even more self-centred. Because her chakras were blocked, nothing was getting in or out physically or emotionally. I saw her as trapped in a tunnel that she had got into. With a little help from me she was going to have to get out.

I investigated the use of the Bach flower remedies and advised her to buy Elm, which helps a person to get back their resolve. This proved to be a very successful healing. It was purely a psychological and emotional condition. There were no Spirits or geopathic stress.

ELECTRICAL RAYS

A CLIENT who was in need of my help sent me a plan of their property. I found it was an almost impossible situation as far as geopathic stress was concerned. Electrical rays from the road lighting were coming straight into this flat. There was also a mobile phone tower of very high intensity.

I did my best to clear as much as I could. Sometimes I can improve a situation but not as much as I would like. When you have geopathic stress it's not the same as having a presence in the house, and you're inclined to feel unwell or very tired. With discarnates, the energy often makes you feel uneasy or depressed. When a client tells me how they are feeling I can more or less guess what the problem is.

A WIDOW

A WOMAN from Dorset contacted me for help. She was a spiritualist. She went to spiritualist meetings and had done so all her life. After she had been widowed for some time, unusual things started happening in her bedroom at night. She thought it was her husband's Spirit. The lights would go off and on at night and the lampshades started moving and rattling around.

I couldn't accept that her husband would really want to make her nervous and upset. She used to contact her husband at spiritualist meetings through mediums, and she wasn't aware that this presence in her bedroom could be something less affectionate.

I investigated and found she had five discarnates around her of the kind which meant that, under their influence, she wasn't really thinking things through properly. They were damaging her judgement. She was also having a problem with her daughter, and was a bit low anyway, because of family issues, so these Thought Forms (an energy which can affect a person's clarity, their reasonable judgement) had more of a chance of getting to her. And she was lonely. She had been widowed a few years and I think these Thought Forms had been around since her bereavement. I cleared the discarnates and gave healing to her and her daughter. She rang after a few weeks, saying she felt much better – but her lampshade had started moving again! She had a real fixation about it being the Spirit of her husband, which it was not! He had been drawn back umpteen times at meetings and he hadn't been allowed to move on. She *wanted* him there, really.

But this was something far worse than the Thought Forms that had been around, and a serious problem was manifesting. It was a poltergeist. It was destructive – things started to be hurled across the bedroom.

In order to calm her down, I suggested she sleep in the spare room with a light on, or a candle, for about a month. After she moved bedrooms I managed to clear the poltergeist, and my client felt totally different. Her vibration returned to normal.

Often poltergeists just want to be released, and therefore they need to make their presence felt. Once the Spirit went away it was as though I'd given the house a spring clean. Nothing like that ever happened again in this lady's lifetime. The Thought Forms had come to her in her bereavement. I think going to meetings hoping to get messages from her husband was partly to blame. She was unwilling to believe that these contacts have to end at some point. Not only did I use my symbols for this healing, but also a rosary which had been blessed. I have used this several times, and it is most effective. This client was an elderly lady and I felt sorry for her, but she had been unable to draw a line under her husband's death.

I have another client who thinks her deceased father is around. I asked through the pendulum if this was the case, and it definitely isn't her father, but she could not accept this. And as long as she *thinks* it is, she has an open door for lost Spirits to come in for comfort. It's very important to draw a line under someone's death. This is where Bereavement Counselling comes in. You are helped to get over the loss and to move on.

BLACK ENERGY

THERE IS a form of energy called Black Energy. Black Energies are man-made and are formed from people's negative thoughts and actions. If somebody has led a really bad life and they die in this state they leave the equivalent of a poisonous fog behind. It's not the same as sudden death. It's like dying in a guilty state or a state of sin. The soul goes to God, but this Black Energy can be left behind.

It is possible to clear this energy with certain symbols. We don't want to send this energy to God, so where do we send it? We have to send it to the nether world where it does not interfere with man nor beast. If we look at places like cemeteries and hospitals, there are undoubtedly quite a number of people there who have died in that condition. We can detect that Black Energy is around with a pendulum, and it is like a black cloud hanging over someone, sometimes since birth.

Earthbound Spirits are not invited in by people, but stay around on the earth plane for a number of years (so I'm told) and then they ascend to the astral plane and this actually is not too far above our ground level. So there is a whole place here, a parallel world that we do not see. They stay there waiting to go to their spiritual home and we can help them with the pendulum, prayer and meditation.

On the astral plane there isn't really time as we know it. How long Spirits stay around depends on the circumstances in which people die and how unwilling they are to move on.

Some discarnates may not even realise they are dead. Some are unwilling to move on and leave loved ones behind. They might carry guilt and be afraid of being punished. I think that's why we often get such simplistic messages through mediums, very often because there's nothing to say. Sometimes you are fortunate enough to get a message that is deep and spiritual and philosophical. But not always. All this does explain how somebody who doesn't know they are dead or who doesn't want to move on can, perhaps through their own wishes and desires, not go to the astral plane. That's the reason why ghosts are walking around for hundreds of years. This is the Imprint of their life. They walk up these steps (that aren't there any more) and float along corridors that were long ago demolished.

Black Energy is a residue that gets left behind, rather like rubbish at a picnic. It's spiritual pollution.

IMPRINTS

ONE OF my clients always seemed to have terrible problems when moving furniture in and out of property. I dowsed and discovered there was an Imprint connected with possessions (an Imprint, in my work, is a trait that has been established during personal trauma, or handed down from previous generations). Very negative energy from a deceased grandmother had left this Imprint on various women in the family – daughter-in-law, granddaughter and great granddaughter. This Imprint was like a footprint in the sand that hadn't been washed away by the tide. I felt that my client was still holding on to an overspill of unhappiness from her mother's past. The experiences were as real as if they had only happened last week, not sixty years ago. *Her* mother had been forced to move into her mother-in-law's house after her marriage because her own home had been bombed during the Blitz. This had been a horrendous experience that had caused her to have a nervous breakdown.

When my client's father retired they had moved into a beautiful home near the sea. But certain aspects of her mother's personality and past still hadn't been resolved. Through the medium of the pendulum, I 'looked' at the house. It had an Imprint that needed clearing: a medium-strength, negative force that would attract unhappy Spirits. Although the grandmother hadn't lived in the house she was around spiritually. She wasn't haunting anybody but was stamping her nature on whoever was receptive. My client's mother, younger sister and daughter were all vulnerable. Her sister wasn't possessed but could *behave* just like her grandmother. She became controlling, nasty and very impulsive. She wasn't like that all the time and certainly didn't have any personal issues with her grandmother. She had been a baby when the grandmother died. However, she was open (spiritually) to the influence of this Imprint, taking on and showing the negative side of her grandmother.

This bad force was very strong. The granddaughter took after her aunt and was also open to the influence of her great-grandmother. There had been difficulties and arguments *every time* furniture was moved. Removal men had suddenly become very unpleasant and unpredictable because of the influence of the grandmother's Spirit, which wanted to interfere with every new venture. Half a century after her death the grandmother's influence over the family was still top of the scale. She had been a dominating woman who had always worn black. Her daughter-in-law had been afraid of her. She still wanted to cause difficulties. The arguments over the furniture and the upsetting removals were occasions that she could influence and control. Some Spirits move lampshades or take pictures down. This one created upsets.

I used a symbol that is effective when dealing with powerful negative forces. I asked the grandmother if she wanted to be released from her earthbound life. She did. I asked her to go to the Light of God and sent her up with love. She seemed to have lacked the love she needed in her own life, either from her parents or her husband. She wanted to go – but it was a struggle. There were two sides to her. She could be nice and easygoing but her other side wasn't pleasant. She was meddlesome. As an earthbound Spirit, she found that she could still control people and that's why she really didn't want to go. I put a healing light around her.

This Spirit was like somebody sitting in a chair, thinking about getting up but not actually moving! She very slowly made up her mind to leave, but it was difficult.

My client was emotionally neutral and hadn't been personally influenced by her grandmother, but often became a victim of the negative influence exerted on other family members. After my client's father died her sister became very domineering. When her mother died she had experienced tremendous difficulty sorting out the estate because of her sister's irrational behaviour. Grandmother had been able to influence my client's sister and her own daughter because, although both sometimes showed great determination, on other occasions they showed very little control over their feelings and actions. The daughter manifested the influence through being dominating and angry. I didn't pick up Greed, although you might expect it with quarrels over possessions. However, there was a Sense of Injustice, also Moodiness and Resentment. Both sister and daughter were carrying this with them as part of their life Programmes. I cleared these negative traits (although it may not be permanent) and gave them both healing. If they respond to the effects of the clearing – i.e. become more kindly and positive – they have a good chance of having much better relationships in and out of family life. I also gave a healing to my client, who badly needed it after recounting this very long saga.

My client's father had repeated the parenting he had received from his dominating mother. He, in turn, was against her career choice and choice of husband. Both he and her sister had refused to attend the wedding. My client felt that some of that was still blocking her progress. She wanted to be free but felt that unconsciously she was holding herself back. She felt as if she had been strangled, controlled by something around her. She had spent a lot of time alone and become much more aware of this feeling.

I cleared more negativity and got her to imagine she was in a bubble of spiritual protection. With psychological damage you have to heal the mind. It is wrong for someone to be dominated by a parent's behaviour for the whole of their life. This has to be worked through by realising it is irrational and they can do whatever they choose. If the grandmother had still been alive she would have been laying down the law.

I closed the healing by asking that any move or any future situation that might be difficult, or 'loaded', would be defused.

A FINE LINE

THERE IS a fine line between an acute case of spiritual negativity and simply a personality or environmental problem. If there is a change in the atmosphere of a home or if people start acting in a way that is 'out of sync' with their normal personality – particularly if it's upsetting – I think this should be investigated.

Teenagers are particularly vulnerable. When they are taking drugs and alcohol it is very easy for Spirits to hang around and influence their behaviour. A drug addict or a young person who is taking drugs on a regular basis nearly always has a discarnate around them. When there is a group, these Spirits hang around like people who have missed the bus! We talk about our shadow side, the slightly dark side that can be easily inhabited by Spirits. Spirits get into auras quite easily if people are weak and lack protection.

If I find any Spirits in an aura I know this is bound to have an impact on someone's behaviour. It might not be serious, but it is enough to knock people off balance emotionally. If someone is considering seeking the help of a therapist, then it would probably be a good idea to consult someone like myself initially so that we can clear away as much of the negativity as possible before they go for treatment. If somebody has a rash or sore you have to cleanse the area before treatment. After a spiritual cleansing it is easier for the therapist or psychiatrist to observe a client's true personal traits and their problems.

The extent of this form of 'clearing' can reach beyond the spiritual, and recently I have been asked to involve myself in clearing blocks preventing house sales and business purchases, with very successful results.

I am probably just scratching the surface of the power we have to transform ourselves and our society. The revelation continues...

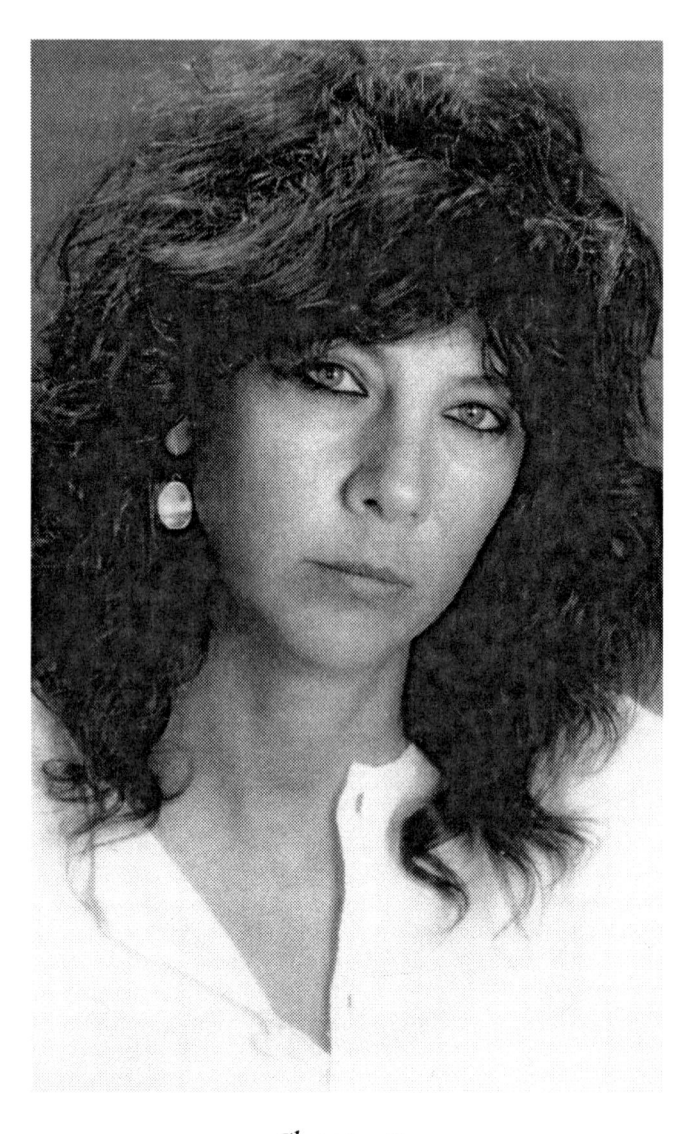

Christine Day

Printed in the United Kingdom by
Lightning Source UK Ltd., Milton Keynes
141815UK00001B/26/A

9 781844 016914